The Lyme Disease Solution

A Holistic Guide to Preventing and Healing from Lyme Disease

Dr Emily John

COPYRIGHT PAGE

TABLE OF CONTENTS

INTRODUCTION

Lyme disease is a debilitating and often misunderstood condition that affects thousands of people worldwide. It is caused by the bacterium Borrelia burgdorferi and is transmitted to humans through the bite of infected black-legged ticks. Despite its prevalence, many people are still unfamiliar with the symptoms and effects of Lyme disease, making it a complex and often challenging condition to diagnose and treat.

Lyme disease was first recognized in 1975 and is named after the town of Lyme, Connecticut where a cluster of cases was identified. Since then, the disease has spread to become a global concern, with reported cases in North America, Europe, and Asia. The number of cases has continued to rise in recent years, with the Centers for Disease Control and

Prevention (CDC) estimating that over 300,000 people are diagnosed with Lyme disease each year in the United States alone.

The symptoms of Lyme disease can range from mild to severe and can be difficult to identify as they often mimic other conditions such as the flu or other viral infections. Some of the most common symptoms include fatigue, fever, headache, muscle and joint aches, and a bull's-eye shaped rash around the site of the tick bite. In some cases, the symptoms may not appear for several weeks or even months after the bite, making it difficult for individuals to link their symptoms to the tick bite.

If left untreated, Lyme disease can progress to later stages and can cause more serious health problems such as memory problems, joint and muscle pain, and neurological symptoms such as facial palsy and meningitis. In severe cases, the disease can cause permanent damage to the heart, nervous system, and other organs, leading to long-term health complications.

One of the biggest challenges of Lyme disease is the lack of clear and consistent diagnostic tests. Currently, the most commonly used test for Lyme disease is the enzyme-linked immunosorbent assay (ELISA), which is a blood test that measures the presence of antibodies to the Borrelia bacterium. However, the ELISA test is not always accurate, and false negatives are not uncommon, making it difficult for individuals to receive a definitive diagnosis.

Treatment for Lyme disease can also be difficult, as the bacteria can be difficult to eradicate from the body. The standard treatment for early-stage Lyme disease is antibiotics, which are typically administered for a period of two to four weeks. However, for some individuals, antibiotics may not be enough to fully eliminate the bacteria, leading to persistent symptoms and ongoing health problems.

There is growing interest in alternative and holistic approaches to the treatment of Lyme disease, including the use of dietary changes, herbal supplements, and mind-body therapies such as meditation and yoga. These approaches aim to support the body's natural healing processes and strengthen the immune system to help the body fight the bacterium.

While conventional medicine has a role to play in the treatment of Lyme disease, it is important to consider all available options and find the best approach for each individual. A holistic approach can help individuals with Lyme disease take control of their health, reduce their symptoms, and improve their quality of life.

Importance of a Holistic Approach

In today's fast-paced world, people are often caught up in the hustle and bustle of daily life and neglect their health and wellbeing. Many people are turning to quick-fix solutions to alleviate their symptoms, rather than taking a more holistic approach to their health.

A holistic approach to health and wellness involves considering all aspects of an individual's life and taking a proactive, rather than reactive, approach to maintaining health and preventing illness. This approach considers the body, mind, and spirit as interconnected, and recognizes that all aspects of an individual's life impact their overall health and wellbeing.

One of the key benefits of a holistic approach to health is that it allows individuals to address the root causes of their health issues, rather than just treating symptoms. For example, if a person is experiencing chronic pain, a conventional approach would likely involve pain medication or other drugs to alleviate the symptoms.

However, this approach does not address the underlying cause of the pain, which could be due to factors such as stress, poor nutrition, or a sedentary lifestyle. A holistic approach, on the other hand, would address all of these factors and strive to find the root cause of the pain in order to help the person achieve lasting relief.

Another key benefit of a holistic approach to health is that it allows individuals to take control of their own health and wellbeing. Many people feel disempowered by the healthcare system, and feel that they are at the mercy of their doctors. A holistic approach encourages individuals to become active participants in their own health and wellness, and empowers them to make informed choices about their own care. This can lead to greater satisfaction with the healthcare experience and better outcomes.

In addition to the benefits for individuals, a holistic approach to health also has significant benefits for society as a whole. This approach recognizes that health is not just the absence of disease, but is a complex interplay of physical, mental, and spiritual factors. By addressing all of these factors, a holistic approach has the potential to reduce healthcare costs, as individuals are more likely to stay healthy and avoid chronic illness.

One of the key components of a holistic approach to health is nutrition. A healthy diet is essential for maintaining good health and preventing disease. A holistic approach recognizes that different people have different nutritional needs, and that what works for one person may not work for another.

For example, a person with a gluten intolerance may need to avoid gluten in their diet, while another person may thrive on a diet rich in carbohydrates. A holistic approach to nutrition involves working with an individual to find the right diet for their unique needs, and making changes as needed to support optimal health.

Another key component of a holistic approach to health is physical activity. Regular exercise is essential for maintaining good health and preventing disease. A holistic approach recognizes that different people have different physical needs, and that what works for one person may not work for another. For example, a person with joint pain may need to avoid high-impact exercises, while another person may thrive on a regular running routine. A holistic approach to physical activity involves working with an individual to find the right exercise program for their unique needs, and making changes as needed to support optimal health.

Chapter 1: Understanding Lyme Disease

Causes and Risk Factors

Lyme disease is an infectious condition caused by the Borrelia bacteria, which is transmitted to humans through the bite of infected black-legged ticks. While it is a relatively new disease, first identified in the 1970s, it has become a growing concern due to the increasing number of cases being reported worldwide. In order to effectively prevent and treat Lyme disease, it is important to understand its causes and risk factors.

The Borrelia bacteria that causes Lyme disease is primarily found in the digestive systems of infected ticks, which feed on the blood of small mammals, birds, and humans. When a tick bites a person, it releases the bacteria into the person's bloodstream, where it begins to multiply and spread throughout the body.

One of the main causes of Lyme disease is exposure to infected ticks. This can occur in a variety of ways, including spending time in wooded or grassy areas, participating in outdoor activities such as camping or hiking, or even just gardening in your own backyard. Ticks are most commonly found in areas with dense vegetation, and are most active during the spring and summer months when temperatures are warm.

Another cause of Lyme disease is the lack of preventive measures to reduce the risk of tick bites. This can include not wearing protective clothing when spending time outdoors, failing to use insect repellent, and not performing regular tick checks after spending time in areas where ticks are present.

In addition to exposure to infected ticks, there are several other risk factors that can increase the likelihood of developing Lyme disease. These include:

- Living in or traveling to areas with a high incidence of Lyme disease, such as the Northeast and Upper Midwest regions of the United States, as well as certain areas of Europe and Asia.

- Having a weakened immune system, which makes it more difficult for the body to fight off the infection.

- Engaging in outdoor activities in areas with high tick populations, such as camping, hiking, or gardening.

- Being over 50 years of age, as the risk of Lyme disease increases with age.

- Having a history of tick bites, as repeated exposure increases the risk of developing the disease.

It is important to understand that not everyone who is bitten by an infected tick will develop Lyme disease. However, the risk of developing the disease increases with the length of time that a tick is attached to the skin and feeding on the person's blood.

Symptoms and Diagnosis

Lyme disease is a complex and multi-systemic illness that can cause a wide range of symptoms. Its diagnosis can often be difficult because the symptoms can mimic those of other conditions, leading to misdiagnosis or delayed treatment. Understanding the symptoms and diagnosis of Lyme disease is important for those at risk of contracting the disease and for those who may already be suffering from it.

Symptoms of Lyme disease can be divided into three stages: early, late and long-term. The early stage of Lyme disease is characterized by the appearance of a bull's-eye rash, also known as erythema migrans, as well as flu-like symptoms such as fever, headache, fatigue, muscle and joint aches, and swollen lymph nodes. In some cases, there may be no rash or only a small, barely noticeable rash.

If left untreated, Lyme disease can progress to the late stage, where it can cause more serious symptoms such as neurocognitive problems, joint and muscle pain, and cardiovascular problems. In the late stage, Lyme disease can also cause more serious symptoms such as memory loss, confusion, depression, and sleep disturbances.

Long-term Lyme disease can result in chronic symptoms, including fatigue, joint and muscle pain, neurocognitive problems, and other persistent symptoms. In some cases, these symptoms can persist for years, even after the initial infection has been treated.

Diagnosing Lyme disease can be challenging, as the symptoms can be similar to those of other conditions. In many cases, a physician may perform a physical examination and take a patient's medical history to determine if they may have Lyme disease. In addition, laboratory testing may be performed to confirm the diagnosis.

The most commonly used laboratory test for Lyme disease is the enzyme-linked immunosorbent assay (ELISA) test, which is designed to detect antibodies to the bacteria that cause Lyme disease. If the ELISA test is positive, it may be followed by a western blot test, which is designed to confirm the presence of Lyme disease antibodies.

In some cases, the ELISA and western blot tests may be negative, even in patients who have clear symptoms of Lyme disease. In these cases, other diagnostic tests, such as a polymerase chain reaction (PCR) test or a culture test, may be used to identify the presence of the Lyme disease bacterium in a patient's blood or body fluid.

In addition to laboratory testing, a physician may also use imaging tests, such as an X-ray, MRI, or CT scan, to help diagnose Lyme disease. These tests may be used to identify any joint damage or other physical abnormalities that may be associated with the disease.

It is important to note that some patients with Lyme disease may not have any symptoms at all, or may only have mild symptoms that do not interfere with their daily activities. In these cases, a physician may not diagnose Lyme disease until much later, when more serious symptoms develop.

Stages of Lyme Disease

The first stage of Lyme disease is referred to as the early localized stage and usually occurs within a few days to several weeks after a tick bite. During this stage, a characteristic bull's eye rash may appear at the site of the bite, along with flu-like symptoms such as fever, fatigue, headache, muscle aches, and joint pain. Some people may not even notice a rash, but the symptoms are still present.

The second stage of Lyme disease is called the early disseminated stage and occurs several weeks to months after the initial infection. During this stage, the bacteria have spread from the site of the bite to other parts of the body, such as the heart, nervous system, and joints. As a result, new symptoms may develop, including heart palpitations, difficulty concentrating, memory loss, numbness or tingling in the limbs, and joint swelling.

The late disseminated stage of Lyme disease is also referred to as chronic Lyme disease and can occur months to years after the initial infection. During this stage, the bacteria have spread even further and may have affected many parts of the body.

This can cause long-lasting symptoms such as chronic fatigue, muscle and joint pain, memory and concentration problems, and depression. In some cases, Lyme disease can cause severe neurological symptoms, such as Bell's palsy, meningitis, or even memory loss.

It is important to note that not all people with Lyme disease will experience all of these stages and the symptoms can vary greatly from person to person. In some cases, the disease may be difficult to diagnose and misdiagnosis is common, leading to delayed or inadequate treatment. This is why it is essential for healthcare providers to be knowledgeable about the different stages of Lyme disease and to use a combination of clinical and laboratory tests to make an accurate diagnosis.

Treatment for Lyme disease depends on the stage of the disease and the symptoms that are present. In the early stages, antibiotics are usually effective in treating the infection and preventing it from spreading. However, in the later stages, treatment can be more challenging and may involve a combination of antibiotics, anti-inflammatory drugs, and alternative therapies such as acupuncture or herbal remedies.

It is also important for people with Lyme disease to adopt a healthy lifestyle, including a balanced diet, regular exercise, stress management techniques, and a strong support system. In some cases, people with chronic Lyme disease may also benefit from rehabilitation therapy to help them regain strength and improve their quality of life.

Chapter 2: Prevention

Avoiding Tick Bites

Lyme disease is a growing problem in many parts of the world, and it's becoming more and more important to take steps to prevent tick bites. Ticks are tiny insects that can carry the bacterium responsible for Lyme disease, and they can be found in many different environments, including forests, fields, and even suburban yards.

If you're planning on spending time outdoors this summer, it's important to be aware of the risks of tick bites and to take steps to protect yourself. In this article, we'll take a closer look at ticks, the diseases they can carry, and what you can do to avoid tick bites.

Understanding Ticks

Ticks are small, spider-like creatures that feed on the blood of animals and humans. They are typically found in wooded or grassy areas, and they're most active during the warm months of the year.

Ticks can be very small, making them difficult to spot. They are also very good at hiding, often clinging to the tips of leaves or blades of grass, where they can wait for a passing host. Once they've found a suitable host, they will latch on and feed until they're full.

Ticks are a major health concern because they can carry a number of different diseases, including Lyme disease, Rocky Mountain spotted fever, and babesiosis. These diseases can cause serious health problems, so it's important to take steps to prevent tick bites.

Preventing Tick Bites

There are a number of steps you can take to avoid tick bites, including:

- Wearing protective clothing: When you're spending time in areas where ticks are present, it's important to wear long-sleeved shirts and pants to help protect your skin. Light-colored clothing can also make it easier to spot any ticks that may be on you.

- Using insect repellent: Insect repellent can help keep ticks away, and there are many different options available, including sprays, lotions, and even wristbands. Be sure to choose an insect repellent that contains DEET, which is the most effective ingredient for preventing tick bites.

- Checking your body regularly: Ticks can be very small, so it's important to check your body regularly for any signs of bites. This is especially important if you've been spending time in areas where ticks are present. Be sure to check your entire body, including your hair, armpits, and the back of your legs.

- Staying on well-trodden paths: When you're hiking or walking in areas where ticks are present, it's a good idea to stay on well-trodden paths to avoid coming into contact with tall grass and other areas where ticks may be hiding.

- Keeping your lawn well-trimmed: Ticks need tall grass and other vegetation to thrive, so it's a good idea to keep your lawn well-trimmed to help reduce the risk of tick bites.

Removing Ticks

If you do find a tick on your body, it's important to remove it as quickly as possible to reduce the risk of disease transmission. To remove a tick, you should:

- Use fine-tipped tweezers: Gently grasp the tick as close to the skin as possible and pull straight out. Don't twist the tick or use a match or other heat source to try to remove it, as this can increase the risk of disease transmission.

- Clean the area: After removing the tick, be sure to clean the bite area thoroughly with soap and water.

- Watch for symptoms: If you've been bitten by a tick, be sure to monitor yourself for any signs of illness, including fever, fatigue, and a bull's-eye rash. If you experience any symptoms, be sure to see a doctor as soon as possible.

Strengthening the Immune System

Strengthening the immune system is an essential aspect of overall health and wellness. Our immune system is responsible for protecting us from harmful pathogens and diseases, and when it is functioning optimally, it can prevent us from getting sick. Unfortunately, our immune system can become weakened due to various factors such as stress, lack of sleep, poor diet, and exposure to toxins.

The good news is that there are several simple and effective ways to boost our immune system and improve our overall health. Here are some strategies that you can implement to improve your immune system and reduce your risk of illness and disease:

1. Eating a healthy and balanced diet: Our diet plays a crucial role in shaping our immune system and overall health. A diet that is rich in nutrients, vitamins, and minerals can help to strengthen the immune system and reduce the risk of illness. Eating a variety of fruits and vegetables, whole grains, lean proteins, and healthy fats is essential for providing our

bodies with the nutrients it needs to function optimally.

2. Reducing stress: Stress is a major factor in weakening our immune system. When we are stressed, our body releases cortisol, a hormone that can suppress our immune system. To reduce stress, try to incorporate stress-reducing activities into your daily routine, such as yoga, meditation, deep breathing, or exercise.

3. Getting enough sleep: Sleep is essential for our overall health, including our immune system. When we don't get enough sleep, our body's ability to fight off illness and disease can be significantly impacted. Aim to get between 7-9 hours of sleep each night to help your body and immune system function optimally.

4. Exercise regularly: Exercise is another important aspect of maintaining a healthy immune system. Physical activity can help to

reduce stress and improve circulation, which can boost the immune system. Aim to exercise for at least 30 minutes each day, and consider incorporating a variety of physical activities such as cardio, strength training, and yoga.

5. Reducing exposure to toxins: Our environment is filled with toxins, such as pollutants and chemicals, that can weaken our immune system. To reduce exposure to toxins, try to avoid using chemical-based products, such as cleaning products, personal care items, and processed foods. Instead, opt for natural and organic products whenever possible.

6. Supplements and herbs: Certain supplements and herbs can also help to boost the immune system and prevent illness. For example, echinacea, garlic, and ginger are all known for their immune-boosting properties. Consult with a healthcare provider to

determine which supplements and herbs may be right for you.

7. Staying hydrated: Drinking enough water is crucial for maintaining a healthy immune system. When we are dehydrated, our body's ability to fight off illness and disease can be compromised. Aim to drink at least 8 glasses of water each day, and consider incorporating herbal teas and fresh juices into your diet.

Holistic Lifestyle Changes

In today's fast-paced and stressful world, more and more people are realizing the importance of taking a holistic approach to their health and well-being. Holistic living is about taking care of the whole person—mind, body, and spirit—rather than just focusing on physical symptoms or health problems. By making holistic lifestyle changes, individuals can improve their overall health, increase energy levels, reduce stress, and achieve a greater sense of balance and well-being.

One of the keys to a holistic lifestyle is recognizing the interconnectedness of all aspects of our lives. Our physical health is directly related to our emotional, mental, and spiritual health, and vice versa. By making positive changes in one area of our lives, we can improve our overall well-being and see benefits in many other areas as well.

One of the first steps in making holistic lifestyle changes is to examine our current habits and practices. This may involve looking at what we eat, how we exercise, how we manage stress, and how we spend our time. It's important to take a critical look at what is working well and what needs improvement, and then make changes that align with our goals and values.

Nutrition is a critical aspect of holistic living. A balanced and nutritious diet can help improve physical health, reduce the risk of chronic diseases, increase energy levels, and support mental and emotional well-being. In contrast, a diet that is high in processed foods, sugar, and unhealthy fats can contribute to a range of health problems and negatively impact our overall well-being.

To support optimal health, it is important to eat a variety of whole, nutrient-dense foods, such as fruits and vegetables, lean proteins, whole grains, and healthy fats. It's also important to limit or eliminate processed foods, sugar, and unhealthy fats from our diets.

Exercise is another key component of a holistic lifestyle. Regular physical activity can help improve physical health, reduce stress, boost mood, and support overall well-being. It is recommended that individuals aim for at least 30 minutes of moderate-intensity physical activity each day, such as brisk walking, cycling, or swimming. It's also important to incorporate a variety of physical activities into our routine, such as strength training, yoga, and stretching, to help keep our bodies strong, flexible, and balanced.

Stress management is another important aspect of holistic living. Chronic stress can have a significant impact on our physical and mental health, and can contribute to a range of health problems, including depression, anxiety, and heart disease. To manage stress, it's important to engage in stress-reducing activities, such as exercise, meditation, deep breathing, and spending time in nature. It's also important to identify and address the sources of stress in our lives and make changes to reduce its impact.

In addition to making changes in our diets, exercise habits, and stress management practices, it's also important to make time for self-care and relaxation. This may include engaging in hobbies, spending time with friends and family, and taking time for quiet reflection and meditation. By making time for self-care, we can reduce stress, boost our mood, and improve our overall well-being.

Finally, it's important to create a supportive environment that promotes holistic living. This may involve seeking out like-minded individuals, joining a supportive community, and making changes in our home and work environments that align with our goals and values. By creating a supportive environment, we can make it easier to stick to our holistic lifestyle changes and achieve our goals.

Chapter 3: Conventional Treatment

Antibiotic Therapy

Antibiotic therapy is a critical component of conventional treatment for Lyme disease. Antibiotics are drugs that target and destroy bacteria, and they are often prescribed to patients with Lyme disease in order to eliminate the Lyme-causing bacteria, Borrelia burgdorferi.

While antibiotics can be effective in treating early-stage Lyme disease, they are not a cure-all solution. It is important to understand the limitations and potential side effects of antibiotics, as well as the role they play in a comprehensive approach to treating Lyme disease.

Antibiotic therapy for Lyme disease is usually a multi-step process that involves several different antibiotics. In the early stages of Lyme disease, a single round of antibiotics is often enough to eliminate the bacteria and cure the infection. However, in more advanced cases, patients may require multiple rounds of antibiotics over a longer period of time. In some cases, patients with persistent symptoms may need to take antibiotics for several months or even years.

The first-line antibiotics for Lyme disease are doxycycline, amoxicillin, and cefuroxime axetil. Doxycycline is a tetracycline antibiotic that is effective against a wide range of bacteria, including the Lyme-causing bacteria. Amoxicillin is a penicillin-like antibiotic that is also effective against a wide range of bacteria, and cefuroxime axetil is a cephalosporin antibiotic that is also used to treat Lyme disease.

Antibiotics can have a range of side effects, and these side effects can be more pronounced in patients with Lyme disease who are taking antibiotics for extended periods of time. Common side effects of antibiotics include gastrointestinal symptoms, such as nausea, vomiting, and diarrhea. Antibiotics can also cause skin rashes, headaches, and other symptoms. In rare cases, antibiotics can cause severe side effects, such as liver damage, anaphylaxis, and other allergic reactions.

While antibiotics are an important part of conventional treatment for Lyme disease, they are not a cure-all solution. Antibiotics do not always eliminate the Lyme-causing bacteria completely, and in some cases, the bacteria can persist even after multiple rounds of antibiotics. This persistence of bacteria is referred to as post-treatment Lyme disease syndrome (PTLDS). Patients with PTLDS often experience persistent symptoms, such as fatigue, joint pain, and cognitive impairment, and there is currently no cure for PTLDS.

One of the limitations of antibiotic therapy for Lyme disease is that antibiotics do not address the underlying causes of the disease. Antibiotics only target the bacteria that cause the infection, but they do not address the underlying factors that led to the infection in the first place. For example, antibiotics do not address the underlying issues that led to a weakened immune system, such as poor diet, stress, or exposure to environmental toxins.

In order to address the underlying causes of Lyme disease, a comprehensive approach to treatment is necessary. This approach should involve a combination of conventional and holistic therapies, including antibiotics, nutrition, herbs and supplements, detoxification, and mind-body therapies. By addressing the underlying causes of Lyme disease, patients can improve their chances of achieving a full recovery and avoid the recurrence of symptoms.

Side Effects and Limitations

Conventional treatment for Lyme disease typically involves the use of antibiotics, which can be highly effective in eliminating the infection. However, as with any medical treatment, there are potential side effects and limitations to consider.

One of the most common side effects of antibiotics used to treat Lyme disease is gastrointestinal distress, including nausea, vomiting, and diarrhea. These symptoms can range from mild to severe and may lead to dehydration, electrolyte imbalances, and other complications. Some people may also experience rashes, hives, or other skin reactions as a result of the antibiotics.

Another potential side effect of antibiotics is the disruption of the gut microbiome. The gut microbiome is a complex ecosystem of bacteria and other microorganisms that play a crucial role in maintaining overall health and well-being. Antibiotics can disrupt this delicate balance, leading to a range of issues including bloating, constipation, and reduced immunity. In some cases, the disruption to the gut microbiome can persist even after treatment has been completed, leaving individuals more susceptible to future infections and illnesses.

Additionally, antibiotics can have negative effects on the liver and kidneys, potentially causing damage or impairing their ability to function properly. In rare cases, antibiotics can also cause serious allergic reactions, including anaphylaxis, a potentially life-threatening condition that requires immediate medical attention.

One of the most significant limitations of conventional treatment for Lyme disease is that it does not address the underlying causes of the illness. Antibiotics only eliminate the bacteria causing the infection and do not address the factors that may have led to the individual becoming infected in the first place. This can include underlying health conditions, a weakened immune system, or a lifestyle that is not conducive to overall health and well-being.

Another limitation of conventional treatment is that it does not address the potential long-term effects of Lyme disease, including chronic pain, fatigue, and cognitive impairment. These symptoms may persist even after the infection has been successfully treated, leaving individuals with a reduced quality of life and the need for ongoing medical care and support.

Finally, there is some evidence to suggest that antibiotics may not always be effective in treating Lyme disease, especially in cases where the infection has been present for an extended period of time. In these cases, multiple rounds of antibiotics may be required, or other treatments may be necessary to manage symptoms and promote healing.

Integrating Conventional and Holistic Treatment

Lyme disease is a rapidly spreading illness caused by the bacterium Borrelia burgdorferi, which is transmitted to humans through the bite of infected black-legged ticks. While early diagnosis and treatment can often lead to a full recovery, the disease can cause chronic and debilitating symptoms if left untreated or if the treatment is not effective. As a result, many people affected by Lyme disease are turning to both conventional and holistic treatments in search of relief.

Conventional treatments for Lyme disease typically involve the use of antibiotics, which are often highly effective in the early stages of the disease. However, some patients may experience side effects from the antibiotics, or may not respond well to the treatment. In these cases, alternative therapies and holistic approaches can be extremely beneficial.

Holistic treatments for Lyme disease focus on addressing the root cause of the illness, rather than just treating its symptoms. This approach often involves using natural remedies, such as herbs and supplements, to support the body's natural healing processes. In addition, holistic treatment may also involve lifestyle changes, such as diet modifications, stress reduction techniques, and physical activity, to support overall health and well-being.

Integrating conventional and holistic treatments for Lyme disease can provide the best of both worlds. For example, a patient may begin with a course of antibiotics to address the bacterial infection, and then supplement that treatment with natural remedies to support their immune system and reduce symptoms.

The first step in integrating conventional and holistic treatments is to understand the nature of Lyme disease and the impact it can have on the body. Lyme disease can cause a wide range of symptoms, including joint pain and stiffness, fatigue, muscle weakness, and cognitive difficulties. It can also trigger autoimmune reactions and cause long-term damage to the nervous system, making it important to address both the underlying infection and its symptoms.

One of the key benefits of incorporating holistic treatments into a Lyme disease treatment plan is the ability to reduce the use of antibiotics. This is important because long-term antibiotic use can disrupt the balance of bacteria in the gut, which can contribute to a range of health problems. Holistic treatments, such as probiotics, can help to restore the balance of bacteria in the gut and support overall health.

In addition to supporting the gut microbiome, holistic treatments can also help to reduce inflammation, boost the immune system, and address the root cause of Lyme disease. For example, natural remedies such as turmeric and ginger have been shown to have potent anti-inflammatory effects, and can be effective in reducing joint pain and stiffness.

Herbs and supplements can also be effective in supporting the immune system and reducing symptoms of Lyme disease. For example, the herb Andrographis has been shown to have potent antibacterial properties, and can be helpful in reducing symptoms associated with Lyme disease. In addition, the supplement Vitamin C has been shown to boost the immune system, and can be especially helpful in reducing symptoms during an acute episode of Lyme disease.

In addition to herbs and supplements, diet modifications can also play a key role in integrating conventional and holistic treatments for Lyme disease. A diet that is rich in fresh, whole foods, and low in processed foods and sugar can help to support overall health and reduce symptoms associated with Lyme disease.

Stress reduction techniques, such as yoga and meditation, can also be helpful in reducing symptoms and promoting overall health. These techniques can help to reduce inflammation and promote relaxation, which can be especially beneficial in reducing symptoms associated with Lyme disease.

Finally, it is important to have a strong support system when integrating conventional and holistic treatments for Lyme disease. Support from friends, family, and healthcare professionals can be crucial in helping individuals to navigate their treatment journey and stay motivated. Joining a Lyme disease support group can also be beneficial, as it provides individuals with the opportunity to connect with others who are experiencing similar challenges, and to share information and resources.

Chapter 4: Holistic Healing

The Role of Nutrition

Nutrition plays a crucial role in the prevention and healing of Lyme Disease. A well-balanced and nutritious diet can not only improve the body's immune system, but also help reduce symptoms and support the healing process. In this section, we will discuss the importance of nutrition in Lyme Disease, and the key components that should be included in a diet for those affected by this condition.

First, it is important to understand that Lyme Disease can greatly affect the body's nutritional status. This is because the disease often causes digestive issues, such as nausea, diarrhea, and abdominal pain, which can make it difficult for the body to absorb essential nutrients from food. Additionally, certain medications used to treat Lyme Disease can interfere with the body's ability to absorb certain nutrients, such as calcium, iron, and vitamins B and D.

Given this, it is essential for those with Lyme Disease to focus on getting adequate amounts of key nutrients, such as vitamins, minerals, and antioxidants, through their diet. Here are some of the key components that should be included in a nutritious diet for those with Lyme Disease:

Protein: Protein is essential for building and repairing tissues, as well as producing enzymes, hormones, and immune system molecules. Good sources of protein include lean meats, poultry, fish, eggs, dairy products, and plant-based sources such as beans, legumes, and nuts.

Vitamins and Minerals: Vitamins and minerals play important roles in supporting the immune system, reducing inflammation, and promoting healing. Vitamins C, D, and E, as well as the minerals selenium and zinc, are particularly important for those with Lyme Disease. Foods rich in these nutrients include leafy greens, berries, citrus fruits, sweet potatoes, fatty fish, and nuts and seeds.

Omega-3 Fatty Acids: Omega-3 fatty acids, particularly EPA and DHA, have been shown to have anti-inflammatory effects and to support the immune system. Good sources of omega-3 fatty acids include fatty fish such as salmon and sardines, as well as plant-based sources like flaxseeds and chia seeds.

Probiotics: Probiotics are beneficial bacteria that can help improve gut health and support the immune system. Foods rich in probiotics include fermented foods like yogurt, kefir, and sauerkraut, as well as probiotic supplements.

Antioxidants: Antioxidants are important for reducing oxidative stress and inflammation, which are key factors in the development and progression of Lyme Disease. Foods high in antioxidants include berries, leafy greens, nuts and seeds, and colorful fruits and vegetables.

It is important to note that individual nutritional needs can vary greatly based on factors such as age, gender, and overall health. Therefore, it is recommended that those with Lyme Disease work with a registered dietitian or nutritionist to develop a personalized eating plan that meets their specific needs.

In addition to focusing on key nutrients, it is also important for those with Lyme Disease to avoid certain foods and substances that can be harmful to their health. These include:

Sugar and Processed Foods: High levels of sugar and processed foods can increase inflammation and weaken the immune system. It is best to avoid or limit these foods as much as possible.

Alcohol: Alcohol can interfere with the absorption of certain nutrients, and can also weaken the immune system and increase oxidative stress. It is best to avoid alcohol or limit consumption as much as possible.

Caffeine: Caffeine can increase stress levels and interfere with sleep, which can negatively impact the immune system. It is best to limit or avoid caffeine as much as possible.

Artificial Sweeteners: Artificial sweeteners have been shown to have negative effects on gut health, which can weaken the immune system and increase inflammation. It is best to avoid artificial sweeteners as much as possible and opt for natural sweeteners such as honey or maple syrup instead.

Gluten: For some individuals with Lyme Disease, gluten can cause digestive issues and increase inflammation. It is recommended to avoid gluten or to follow a gluten-free diet if necessary.

Herbs and Supplements

Herbs and supplements have been used for centuries to prevent and treat various health conditions, including Lyme disease. The use of natural remedies has increased in recent years, as people seek alternatives to conventional drugs and treatments that can often have harmful side effects. In this article, we'll explore the role of herbs and supplements in preventing and healing from Lyme disease, and how they can be used as part of a holistic approach to health.

Lyme disease is caused by the bacterium Borrelia burgdorferi, which is transmitted to humans through the bite of infected black-legged ticks. The symptoms of Lyme disease can be varied and range from mild to severe, and if left untreated, the disease can cause long-term health problems. Conventional treatment usually involves antibiotics, which can be effective in early stages of the disease, but they can also cause side effects and are not always effective in treating chronic Lyme disease.

Herbs and supplements can be an effective complement to conventional treatment for Lyme disease. They can help to boost the immune system, reduce inflammation, and provide relief from the symptoms of the disease. Here are some of the most commonly used herbs and supplements for Lyme disease:

1. Olive Leaf Extract: Olive leaf extract is a powerful antioxidant that has anti-inflammatory properties. It has been shown to help fight Lyme disease by reducing the number of Lyme spirochetes in the body and boosting the immune system.

2. Cat's Claw: Cat's claw is an herbal remedy that has been used for centuries to treat various health conditions, including Lyme disease. It is believed to have anti-inflammatory and immune-boosting properties, which makes it a useful tool in the fight against Lyme disease.

3. Andrographis: Andrographis is an herb that has been used in traditional Chinese medicine for thousands of years to treat various health conditions. It has been shown to have antimicrobial and anti-inflammatory properties, which make it a useful tool in the treatment of Lyme disease.

4. Curcumin: Curcumin is a compound found in the spice turmeric, which is a staple ingredient in many Asian dishes. It has been shown to have anti-inflammatory and antioxidant properties, which can help to reduce symptoms of Lyme disease.

5. Japanese Knotweed: Japanese knotweed is an herb that has been used in traditional Chinese medicine for centuries. It is believed to have antimicrobial and anti-inflammatory properties, which make it an effective tool in the treatment of Lyme disease.

6. Vitamin D: Vitamin D is a crucial nutrient that is essential for strong bones and a healthy

immune system. It has been shown to help fight Lyme disease by boosting the immune system and reducing inflammation.

7. Probiotics: Probiotics are beneficial bacteria that live in the gut and help to maintain a healthy digestive system. They have been shown to help boost the immune system, which is important in the fight against Lyme disease.

8. Magnesium: Magnesium is an essential mineral that is required for a healthy immune system. It has been shown to help reduce symptoms of Lyme disease, such as fatigue and muscle pain.

Herbs and supplements can be taken in various forms, including teas, tinctures, capsules, and powders. It is important to speak with a healthcare provider before starting any new treatment, as some herbs and supplements can interact with medications or have other side effects.

Detoxification and Cleansing

Detoxification and cleansing are two essential components of a holistic approach to health and wellness. Our bodies are constantly exposed to a multitude of toxins and pollutants, both from the environment and our diet, that can accumulate and cause a range of health issues. To maintain optimal health and prevent disease, it is important to engage in regular detoxification and cleansing practices to help eliminate these harmful substances.

Detoxification refers to the process of removing toxic substances from the body. This can be achieved through various means, including dietary changes, herbal supplements, and physical activity. Cleansing, on the other hand, is a more comprehensive approach that aims to support the body's natural cleansing processes. A successful cleanse will not only remove toxins, but also support the body's ability to eliminate waste and improve overall health.

There are many benefits to be gained from regular detoxification and cleansing. These practices can help to improve energy levels, boost immunity, support weight loss, and improve mental clarity. They also play an important role in preventing chronic diseases and promoting overall health and wellness.

One of the most effective methods of detoxification is through diet. Eating a diet rich in whole, nutrient-dense foods is essential for supporting the body's natural cleansing processes. This includes consuming plenty of fruits and vegetables, as well as lean protein sources like fish, poultry, and legumes.

These foods are rich in fiber, vitamins, and minerals that help to support the body's natural detoxification processes.

In addition to eating a balanced diet, it is also important to avoid foods that can contribute to the accumulation of toxins in the body. This includes processed foods, sugar, and refined carbohydrates, as well as alcohol and caffeine. These foods can create an acidic environment in the body, which can lead to inflammation and the accumulation of toxins.

Herbs and supplements can also be an effective way to support the body's natural cleansing processes. Milk thistle, for example, has been shown to support liver function and promote the elimination of toxins. Other herbs, such as dandelion root, are known for their diuretic properties and can help to support the elimination of waste through the kidneys.

Additionally, supplements like probiotics can support digestive health and help to eliminate harmful bacteria from the gut.

Physical activity also plays an important role in promoting detoxification. Regular exercise helps to increase circulation and promote the elimination of waste and toxins through the lymphatic system. Engaging in activities like yoga and Tai Chi can also help to reduce stress, which can contribute to the accumulation of toxins in the body.

Cleansing is a more comprehensive approach to detoxification that aims to support the body's natural cleansing processes. This can be achieved through various means, including fasting, juice cleansing, and colon cleansing. Fasting, for example, involves abstaining from solid food for a period of time, allowing the body to focus on eliminating toxins and waste. Juice cleansing involves consuming only fresh fruit and vegetable juices for a set period of time, providing the body with a concentrated source of nutrients and allowing it to focus on cleansing. Colon cleansing, also known as colon hydrotherapy, involves flushing the colon with water to remove waste and promote the elimination of toxins.

Regardless of the method chosen, it is important to approach cleansing with caution. Rapid or extreme cleansing methods can be dangerous and should only be undertaken under the guidance of a healthcare professional. It is also important to remember that cleansing should not be used as a substitute for a balanced diet and regular physical activity. Rather, it should be viewed as a complement to these practices and used in moderation.

Mind-Body Therapies

The mind and body are intimately connected and the health of one can greatly impact the health of the other. This is where mind-body therapies come in, a type of holistic healing practice that recognizes the connection between the mind and body and aims to heal both at the same time. These therapies have been around for centuries and have gained increasing popularity in recent years, especially in the field of holistic health and wellness.

One of the most well-known mind-body therapies is meditation. Meditation is a practice that involves focusing the mind on a particular object, sound, mantra, or the breath. The goal of meditation is to calm the mind and reduce stress, which in turn can improve physical health. There is a growing body of research that supports the benefits of meditation, including reducing symptoms of chronic pain, anxiety, and depression, improving sleep, and reducing blood pressure.

Another popular mind-body therapy is yoga, a practice that involves physical postures, breathing exercises, and meditation. Yoga has been used for thousands of years to improve physical and mental health and is believed to promote balance and harmony in the mind and body. Yoga has been shown to reduce stress, improve flexibility and strength, and boost the immune system.

Breathing exercises, also known as pranayama, are another type of mind-body therapy that can be highly beneficial. Breathing exercises involve controlling the breath in various ways, such as slowing it down or holding it for a certain length of time. Breathing exercises can help to calm the mind, reduce stress and anxiety, and improve physical health by increasing oxygen flow to the body.

Hypnotherapy is another form of mind-body therapy that uses the power of the mind to heal the body. This type of therapy involves inducing a state of deep relaxation and hypnosis, during which the therapist can help the client to change negative thought patterns, overcome fears and phobias, and manage physical symptoms such as pain and anxiety.

Art therapy is another form of mind-body therapy that can be highly beneficial. This type of therapy involves using art, such as drawing, painting, or sculpting, to express emotions and work through personal issues. Art therapy can help to reduce stress and anxiety, improve self-esteem and mood, and promote physical and mental healing.

Finally, guided imagery is another mind-body therapy that can be highly beneficial. Guided imagery involves using visualization and mental imagery to promote physical and mental healing. This type of therapy can be used to manage physical symptoms, reduce stress and anxiety, and improve sleep and mood.

Chapter 5: Coping with Lyme Disease

Managing Symptoms

While Lyme disease is treatable with antibiotics, the disease can cause a wide range of symptoms that can be difficult to manage. In this section, we will explore some of the most common symptoms of Lyme disease and discuss various methods for managing these symptoms.

Joint Pain and Stiffness

Joint pain and stiffness is a common symptom of Lyme disease, and is caused by inflammation in the joints. This inflammation can cause the joints to become swollen, stiff, and painful. To manage joint pain and stiffness, it is important to get plenty of rest and avoid activities that put unnecessary stress on the joints.

Applying heat or ice to the affected joints can also help to relieve pain and stiffness. In addition, gentle exercises such as yoga, tai chi, or walking can help to improve joint flexibility and reduce pain. Over-the-counter pain relievers such as ibuprofen or acetaminophen can also be helpful for managing joint pain and stiffness.

Fatigue

Fatigue is another common symptom of Lyme disease, and can be caused by a number of factors, including anemia, hormonal imbalances, and disruptions in the sleep-wake cycle. To manage fatigue, it is important to get plenty of rest and avoid overexertion. Additionally, incorporating physical activity into your daily routine can help to increase energy levels and reduce fatigue.

Eating a healthy diet that is high in vitamins and minerals can also help to reduce fatigue. Iron-rich foods such as leafy green vegetables, red meat, and poultry can help to prevent anemia, while B-vitamins such as B-12 and folate can help to boost energy levels. Drinking plenty of water can also help to reduce fatigue and improve overall energy levels.

Headaches

Headaches are another common symptom of Lyme disease, and can be caused by a number of factors, including stress, muscle tension, and inflammation. To manage headaches, it is important to practice stress-reducing techniques such as deep breathing, meditation, or yoga.

Over-the-counter pain relievers such as ibuprofen or acetaminophen can also be helpful for managing headaches. In addition, drinking plenty of water and avoiding dehydration can help to reduce headaches, as well as avoiding triggers such as caffeine, alcohol, and processed foods.

Neurological Symptoms

Lyme disease can also cause a range of neurological symptoms, including memory loss, confusion, and difficulty concentrating. To manage these symptoms, it is important to maintain a healthy lifestyle, including eating a balanced diet, getting regular exercise, and getting plenty of rest.

In addition, incorporating activities that stimulate the brain, such as reading, writing, or solving puzzles, can help to improve memory and cognitive function. Using memory aids such as flashcards or note-taking can also be helpful for managing memory loss and improving cognitive function.

Depression and Anxiety

Depression and anxiety are common symptoms of Lyme disease, and can be caused by the physical and emotional impact of the disease. To manage depression and anxiety, it is important to seek support from friends, family, and healthcare providers.

In addition, engaging in activities that promote relaxation and stress-reduction, such as meditation, yoga, or massage, can help to reduce symptoms of depression and anxiety. Incorporating physical activity into your daily routine can also be helpful for managing these symptoms, as exercise has been shown to boost mood and reduce symptoms of depression and anxiety.

Dealing with Emotional Challenges

Life is full of ups and downs, and it can be tough to navigate the rough waters of emotional distress. Whether you're dealing with stress, anxiety, depression, or any other mental health condition, it's essential to understand that these feelings are a normal part of the human experience. However, when these emotions become overwhelming, they can have a significant impact on your life and well-being.

One of the biggest challenges of dealing with emotional difficulties is that they can often feel isolating and embarrassing. You may feel like you're the only one who's struggling or that you should be able to handle your emotions better. It's important to remember that these feelings are common and that you're not alone.

we'll explore some of the most effective strategies for dealing with emotional challenges, including self-care, mindfulness, therapy, and medication.

Self-Care

Self-care is an essential part of dealing with emotional challenges. When you're feeling overwhelmed, it's easy to neglect your own needs and engage in unhealthy coping mechanisms, such as overeating, drinking, or engaging in other harmful behaviors.

To help you manage your emotions, it's crucial to prioritize self-care and make sure that you're taking care of yourself in a healthy way. This can include things like:

- Exercise: Regular physical activity has been shown to have a positive impact on mental health. Whether it's going for a walk, running, or doing yoga, getting your body moving can help you feel better and reduce stress.

- Sleep: Getting enough quality sleep is crucial for managing emotional challenges. Make sure that you're getting enough sleep each night and that you're creating a sleep environment that's conducive to restful sleep.

- Nutrition: Eating a healthy, balanced diet can have a significant impact on your mental health. Make sure that you're eating plenty of fruits and vegetables, whole grains, and lean protein.

- Relaxation: Engaging in relaxation techniques like deep breathing, meditation, or visualization can help you reduce stress and calm your mind.

Mindfulness

Mindfulness is a technique that involves focusing on the present moment and paying attention to your thoughts and feelings without judgment. This can be a powerful tool for managing emotional challenges because it helps you to become more aware of your thoughts and feelings and to develop a greater sense of control over them.

To practice mindfulness, try to set aside time each day to focus on your breath and to become more aware of your thoughts and feelings. You can do this by simply paying attention to the sensation of your breath as you inhale and exhale, or by using guided meditations or visualization exercises.

Therapy

Another effective way to deal with emotional challenges is through therapy. Talking to a mental health professional can help you gain a better understanding of your feelings and provide you with the tools and strategies you need to manage them more effectively.

There are many different types of therapy, including cognitive-behavioral therapy, talk therapy, and psychodynamic therapy, among others. Your therapist will help you choose the best approach for you, based on your specific needs and concerns.

Medication

In some cases, medication may be necessary to help manage emotional challenges. Antidepressants, anxiety medications, and other psychiatric drugs can be effective for some people, but it's important to remember that medication is just one part of a comprehensive approach to managing your emotions.

If you're considering taking medication, it's important to talk to your doctor about the potential benefits and risks and to be honest about any side effects that you experience.

Support from Friends and Family

Support from friends and family is an essential aspect of the healing journey for those with Lyme Disease. The physical, emotional, and psychological challenges that come with this debilitating illness can be overwhelming, but having a supportive network of loved ones can make all the difference. In this chapter, we will explore the different ways in which friends and family can support individuals with Lyme Disease, as well as the importance of maintaining strong relationships during this difficult time.

One of the most critical ways in which friends and family can support someone with Lyme Disease is by being there for them emotionally. This can involve simply listening to their struggles and offering a shoulder to cry on, or it can mean providing encouragement and support when the going gets tough.

For many people with Lyme Disease, the most difficult part of the journey is not neccssarily the physical symptoms, but the emotional toll that the illness takes. The fatigue, brain fog, and joint pain can make it difficult to keep up with daily life, and this can lead to feelings of frustration, anger, and hopelessness. When friends and family offer emotional support and understanding, it can help to alleviate some of these negative emotions and provide comfort during difficult times.

Another way that friends and family can provide support is by helping to manage day-to-day tasks and responsibilities. This can involve anything from grocery shopping and cooking meals to assisting with household chores and transportation.

For those with Lyme Disease, it can be challenging to keep up with their usual routine, and having someone to help out with these tasks can make a big difference. It can also give the individual some much-needed rest and allow them to conserve their energy for healing.

Additionally, friends and family can provide practical support by helping to coordinate appointments and manage medications. This can involve researching different treatments, accompanying the individual to doctor's appointments, and ensuring that medications are taken on schedule. For many people with Lyme Disease, the journey to recovery is a long one, and having someone to help navigate this process can be invaluable.

Having a supportive network of friends and family can also provide a sense of community and connection. This can help to combat feelings of isolation and loneliness that can often accompany Lyme Disease. Being able to talk about the illness and share experiences with others who understand can be incredibly therapeutic, and it can help to build a support system that provides comfort and encouragement.

It is also essential to maintain strong relationships with loved ones during this difficult time. For many people with Lyme Disease, the illness can consume their lives, and they may unintentionally withdraw from those they care about. It is crucial to remember that maintaining relationships with friends and family can provide a much-needed source of comfort and support during this challenging time.

Conclusion

The first step in the path to healing and recovery from Lyme disease is a thorough understanding of the condition. Lyme disease is caused by the bacterium Borrelia burgdorferi, which is transmitted to humans through the bite of infected black-legged ticks.

The symptoms of Lyme disease can range from mild to severe, and can include fatigue, headache, joint pain, muscle aches, and fever. If left untreated, Lyme disease can progress to more serious and chronic stages, leading to a range of debilitating symptoms such as neurological problems, joint pain, and memory loss.

A key component of the path to healing and recovery from Lyme disease is prevention. This involves avoiding exposure to tick bites and taking steps to strengthen the immune system. To reduce the risk of tick bites, it is important to take precautions when spending time outdoors, such as wearing long sleeves and pants and using insect repellent. Additionally, strengthening the immune system can help to reduce the severity of symptoms and improve the body's ability to fight off the infection. This can be done through a healthy diet rich in nutrients, exercise, and stress management techniques.

The next step in the path to healing and recovery from Lyme disease is conventional treatment. Conventional treatment for Lyme disease typically involves a course of antibiotics, which are designed to kill the bacterium responsible for the infection. However, the side effects of antibiotics can be severe, and many people find that they are unable to tolerate the treatment. Additionally, antibiotics can have limited efficacy, particularly in cases of chronic Lyme disease.

To maximize the chances of healing and recovery, it is important to adopt a holistic approach that incorporates both conventional and alternative therapies. This approach should take into account the individual needs and circumstances of each person, and may involve the use of herbs, supplements, and other alternative therapies.

For example, some people find that using herbal remedies like garlic, turmeric, and ginger can help to reduce the severity of symptoms and improve overall health. Additionally, detoxification and cleansing can help to remove toxic substances from the body and promote a healthy immune response.

The final step in the path to healing and recovery from Lyme disease is coping with the emotional challenges that the condition can bring. Lyme disease can be a life-altering condition, and it is not uncommon for people to experience feelings of depression, anxiety, and frustration. It is important to find support from friends, family, and a community of people who understand what you are going through. This can help to provide a sense of comfort and encouragement as you navigate the ups and downs of the healing process.

www.ingramcontent.com/pod-product-compliance
Lightning Source LLC
Chambersburg PA
CBHW070922220526
45467CB00004B/1507